Occupational Safety and Health Act of 1970

"To assure safe and healthful working conditions for working men and women; by authorizing enforcement of the standards developed under the Act; by assisting and encouraging the States in their efforts to assure safe and healthful working conditions; by providing for research, information, education, and training in the field of occupational safety and health."

This guidance is not a standard or regulation, and it creates no new legal obligations. It contains recommendations as well as descriptions of mandatory safety and health standards. The recommendations are advisory in nature, informational in content, and are intended to assist employers in providing a safe and healthful workplace. The Occupational Safety and Health Act requires employers to comply with safety and health standards and regulations promulgated by OSHA or by a state with an OSHA-approved state plan. In addition, the Act's General Duty Clause, Section 5(a)(1), requires employers to provide their employees with a workplace free from recognized hazards likely to cause death or serious physical harm.

This information will be made available to sensory-impaired individuals upon request. Voice phone: (202) 693-1999; teletypewriter (TTY) number: 1-877-889-5627.

Guidance on Preparing Workplaces for COVID-19

U.S. Department of Labor
Occupational Safety and Health Administration

OSHA 3990-03 2020

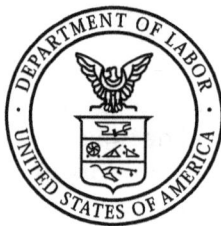

U.S. Department of Labor

Contents

Introduction

Coronavirus Disease 2019 (COVID-19) is a respiratory disease caused by the SARS-CoV-2 virus. It has spread from China to many other countries around the world, including the United States. Depending on the severity of COVID-19's international impacts, outbreak conditions—including those rising to the level of a pandemic—can affect all aspects of daily life, including travel, trade, tourism, food supplies, and financial markets.

To reduce the impact of COVID-19 outbreak conditions on businesses, workers, customers, and the public, it is important for all employers to plan now for COVID-19. For employers who have already planned for influenza pandemics, planning for COVID-19 may involve updating plans to address the specific exposure risks, sources of exposure, routes of transmission, and other unique characteristics of SARS-CoV-2 (i.e., compared to pandemic influenza viruses). Employers who have not prepared for pandemic events should prepare themselves and their workers as far in advance as possible of potentially worsening outbreak conditions. Lack of continuity planning can result in a cascade of failures as employers attempt to address challenges of COVID-19 with insufficient resources and workers who might not be adequately trained for jobs they may have to perform under pandemic conditions.

The Occupational Safety and Health Administration (OSHA) developed this COVID-19 planning guidance based on traditional infection prevention and industrial hygiene practices. It focuses on the need for employers to implement engineering, administrative, and work practice controls and personal protective equipment (PPE), as well as considerations for doing so.

This guidance is intended for planning purposes. Employers and workers should use this planning guidance to help identify risk levels in workplace settings and to determine any appropriate control measures to implement. Additional guidance may be needed as COVID-19 outbreak conditions change, including as new information about the virus, its transmission, and impacts, becomes available.

The U.S. Department of Health and Human Services' Centers for Disease Control and Prevention (CDC) provides the latest information about COVID-19 and the global outbreak: www.cdc.gov/coronavirus/2019-ncov.

The OSHA COVID-19 webpage offers information specifically for workers and employers: www.osha.gov/covid-19.

This guidance is advisory in nature and informational in content. It is not a standard or a regulation, and it neither creates new legal obligations nor alters existing obligations created by OSHA standards or the *Occupational Safety and Health Act* (OSH Act). Pursuant to the OSH Act, employers must comply with safety and health standards and regulations issued and enforced either by OSHA or by an OSHA-approved State Plan. In addition, the OSH Act's General Duty Clause, Section 5(a)(1), requires employers to provide their employees with a workplace free from recognized hazards likely to cause death or serious physical harm. OSHA-approved State Plans may have standards, regulations and enforcement policies that are different from, but at least as effective as, OSHA's. Check with your State Plan, as applicable, for more information.

About COVID-19

Symptoms of COVID-19

Infection with SARS-CoV-2, the virus that causes COVID-19, can cause illness ranging from mild to severe and, in some cases, can be fatal. Symptoms typically include fever, cough, and shortness of breath. Some people infected with the virus have reported experiencing other non-respiratory symptoms. Other people, referred to as *asymptomatic cases*, have experienced no symptoms at all.

According to the CDC, symptoms of COVID-19 may appear in as few as 2 days or as long as 14 days after exposure.

How COVID-19 Spreads

Although the first human cases of COVID-19 likely resulted from exposure to infected animals, infected people can spread SARS-CoV-2 to other people.

The virus is thought to spread mainly from person-to-person, including:

- Between people who are in close contact with one another (within about 6 feet).

- Through respiratory droplets produced when an infected person coughs or sneezes. These droplets can land in the mouths or noses of people who are nearby or possibly be inhaled into the lungs.

Medium exposure risk jobs include those that require frequent and/or close contact with (i.e., within 6 feet of) other people who may be infected with SARS-CoV-2.

It may be possible that a person can get COVID-19 by touching a surface or object that has SARS-CoV-2 on it and then touching their own mouth, nose, or possibly their eyes, but this is not thought to be the primary way the virus spreads.

People are thought to be most contagious when they are most symptomatic (i.e., experiencing fever, cough, and/or shortness of breath). Some spread might be possible before people show symptoms; there have been reports of this type of asymptomatic transmission with this new coronavirus, but this is also not thought to be the main way the virus spreads.

Although the United States has implemented public health measures to limit the spread of the virus, it is likely that some person-to-person transmission will continue to occur.

The CDC website provides the latest information about COVID-19 transmission: www.cdc.gov/coronavirus/2019-ncov/about/transmission.html.

How a COVID-19 Outbreak Could Affect Workplaces

Similar to influenza viruses, SARS-CoV-2, the virus that causes COVID-19, has the potential to cause extensive outbreaks. Under conditions associated with widespread person-to-person spread, multiple areas of the United States and other countries may see impacts at the same time. In the absence of a vaccine, an outbreak may also be an extended event. As a result, workplaces may experience:

- **Absenteeism.** Workers could be absent because they are sick; are caregivers for sick family members; are caregivers for children if schools or day care centers are closed; have at-risk people at home, such as immunocompromised family members; or are afraid to come to work because of fear of possible exposure.

- **Change in patterns of commerce.** Consumer demand for items related to infection prevention (e.g., respirators) is likely to increase significantly, while consumer interest in other goods may decline. Consumers may also change shopping patterns because of a COVID-19 outbreak. Consumers may try to shop at off-peak hours to reduce contact with other people, show increased interest in home delivery services, or prefer other options, such as drive-through service, to reduce person-to-person contact.

- **Interrupted supply/delivery.** Shipments of items from geographic areas severely affected by COVID-19 may be delayed or cancelled with or without notification.

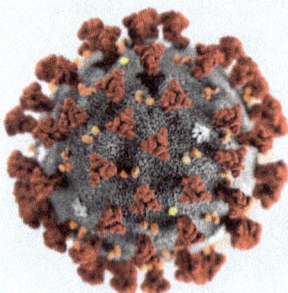

This illustration, created at the Centers for Disease Control and Prevention (CDC), reveals ultrastructural morphology exhibited by the 2019 Novel Coronavirus (2019-nCoV). Note the spikes that adorn the outer surface of the virus, which impart the look of a corona surrounding the virion, when viewed electron microscopically. This virus was identified as the cause of an outbreak of respiratory illness first detected in Wuhan, China.

Photo: CDC / Alissa Eckert & Dan Higgins

Steps All Employers Can Take to Reduce Workers' Risk of Exposure to SARS-CoV-2

This section describes basic steps that every employer can take to reduce the risk of worker exposure to SARS-CoV-2, the virus that causes COVID-19, in their workplace. Later sections of this guidance—including those focusing on jobs classified as having low, medium, high, and very high exposure risks—provide specific recommendations for employers and workers within specific risk categories.

Develop an Infectious Disease Preparedness and Response Plan

If one does not already exist, develop an infectious disease preparedness and response plan that can help guide protective actions against COVID-19.

Stay abreast of guidance from federal, state, local, tribal, and/or territorial health agencies, and consider how to incorporate those recommendations and resources into workplace-specific plans.

Plans should consider and address the level(s) of risk associated with various worksites and job tasks workers perform at those sites. Such considerations may include:

- Where, how, and to what sources of SARS-CoV-2 might workers be exposed, including:
  - The general public, customers, and coworkers; and
  - Sick individuals or those at particularly high risk of infection (e.g., international travelers who have visited locations with widespread sustained (ongoing) COVID-19 transmission, healthcare workers who have had unprotected exposures to people known to have, or suspected of having, COVID-19).
- Non-occupational risk factors at home and in community settings.

- Workers' individual risk factors (e.g., older age; presence of chronic medical conditions, including immunocompromising conditions; pregnancy).
- Controls necessary to address those risks.

Follow federal and state, local, tribal, and/or territorial (SLTT) recommendations regarding development of contingency plans for situations that may arise as a result of outbreaks, such as:

- Increased rates of worker absenteeism.
- The need for social distancing, staggered work shifts, downsizing operations, delivering services remotely, and other exposure-reducing measures.
- Options for conducting essential operations with a reduced workforce, including cross-training workers across different jobs in order to continue operations or deliver surge services.
- Interrupted supply chains or delayed deliveries.

Plans should also consider and address the other steps that employers can take to reduce the risk of worker exposure to SARS-CoV-2 in their workplace, described in the sections below.

Prepare to Implement Basic Infection Prevention Measures

For most employers, protecting workers will depend on emphasizing basic infection prevention measures. As appropriate, all employers should implement good hygiene and infection control practices, including:

- Promote frequent and thorough hand washing, including by providing workers, customers, and worksite visitors with a place to wash their hands. If soap and running water are not immediately available, provide alcohol-based hand rubs containing at least 60% alcohol.
- Encourage workers to stay home if they are sick.
- Encourage respiratory etiquette, including covering coughs and sneezes.

- Provide customers and the public with tissues and trash receptacles.
- Employers should explore whether they can establish policies and practices, such as flexible worksites (e.g., telecommuting) and flexible work hours (e.g., staggered shifts), to increase the physical distance among employees and between employees and others if state and local health authorities recommend the use of social distancing strategies.
- Discourage workers from using other workers' phones, desks, offices, or other work tools and equipment, when possible.
- Maintain regular housekeeping practices, including routine cleaning and disinfecting of surfaces, equipment, and other elements of the work environment. When choosing cleaning chemicals, employers should consult information on Environmental Protection Agency (EPA)-approved disinfectant labels with claims against emerging viral pathogens. Products with EPA-approved emerging viral pathogens claims are expected to be effective against SARS-CoV-2 based on data for harder to kill viruses. Follow the manufacturer's instructions for use of all cleaning and disinfection products (e.g., concentration, application method and contact time, PPE).

Develop Policies and Procedures for Prompt Identification and Isolation of Sick People, if Appropriate

- Prompt identification and isolation of potentially infectious individuals is a critical step in protecting workers, customers, visitors, and others at a worksite.
- Employers should inform and encourage employees to self-monitor for signs and symptoms of COVID-19 if they suspect possible exposure.
- Employers should develop policies and procedures for employees to report when they are sick or experiencing symptoms of COVID-19.

- Where appropriate, employers should develop policies and procedures for immediately isolating people who have signs and/or symptoms of COVID-19, and train workers to implement them. Move potentially infectious people to a location away from workers, customers, and other visitors. Although most worksites do not have specific isolation rooms, designated areas with closable doors may serve as isolation rooms until potentially sick people can be removed from the worksite.

- Take steps to limit spread of the respiratory secretions of a person who may have COVID-19. Provide a face mask, if feasible and available, and ask the person to wear it, if tolerated. Note: A face mask (also called a surgical mask, procedure mask, or other similar terms) on a patient or other sick person should not be confused with PPE for a worker; the mask acts to contain potentially infectious respiratory secretions at the source (i.e., the person's nose and mouth).

- If possible, isolate people suspected of having COVID-19 separately from those with confirmed cases of the virus to prevent further transmission—particularly in worksites where medical screening, triage, or healthcare activities occur, using either permanent (e.g., wall/different room) or temporary barrier (e.g., plastic sheeting).

- Restrict the number of personnel entering isolation areas.

- Protect workers in close contact with (i.e., within 6 feet of) a sick person or who have prolonged/repeated contact with such persons by using additional engineering and administrative controls, safe work practices, and PPE. Workers whose activities involve close or prolonged/repeated contact with sick people are addressed further in later sections covering workplaces classified at medium and very high or high exposure risk.

Develop, Implement, and Communicate about Workplace Flexibilities and Protections

- Actively encourage sick employees to stay home.

- Ensure that sick leave policies are flexible and consistent with public health guidance and that employees are aware of these policies.

- Talk with companies that provide your business with contract or temporary employees about the importance of sick employees staying home and encourage them to develop non-punitive leave policies.

- Do not require a healthcare provider's note for employees who are sick with acute respiratory illness to validate their illness or to return to work, as healthcare provider offices and medical facilities may be extremely busy and not able to provide such documentation in a timely way.

- Maintain flexible policies that permit employees to stay home to care for a sick family member. Employers should be aware that more employees may need to stay at home to care for sick children or other sick family members than is usual.

- Recognize that workers with ill family members may need to stay home to care for them. See CDC's Interim Guidance for Preventing the Spread of COVID-19 in Homes and Residential Communities: www.cdc.gov/coronavirus/2019-ncov/hcp/guidance-prevent-spread.html.

- Be aware of workers' concerns about pay, leave, safety, health, and other issues that may arise during infectious disease outbreaks. Provide adequate, usable, and appropriate training, education, and informational material about business-essential job functions and worker health and safety, including proper hygiene practices and the use of any workplace controls (including PPE). Informed workers who feel safe at work are less likely to be unnecessarily absent.

- Work with insurance companies (e.g., those providing employee health benefits) and state and local health agencies to provide information to workers and customers about medical care in the event of a COVID-19 outbreak.

Implement Workplace Controls

Occupational safety and health professionals use a framework called the "hierarchy of controls" to select ways of controlling workplace hazards. In other words, the best way to control a hazard is to systematically remove it from the workplace, rather than relying on workers to reduce their exposure. During a COVID-19 outbreak, when it may not be possible to eliminate the hazard, the most effective protection measures are (listed from most effective to least effective): engineering controls, administrative controls, safe work practices (a type of administrative control), and PPE. There are advantages and disadvantages to each type of control measure when considering the ease of implementation, effectiveness, and cost. In most cases, a combination of control measures will be necessary to protect workers from exposure to SARS-CoV-2.

In addition to the types of workplace controls discussed below, CDC guidance for businesses provides employers and workers with recommended SARS-CoV-2 infection prevention strategies to implement in workplaces: www.cdc.gov/coronavirus/2019-ncov/specific-groups/guidance-business-response.html.

Engineering Controls

Engineering controls involve isolating employees from work-related hazards. In workplaces where they are appropriate, these types of controls reduce exposure to hazards without relying on worker behavior and can be the most cost-effective solution to implement. Engineering controls for SARS-CoV-2 include:

- Installing high-efficiency air filters.
- Increasing ventilation rates in the work environment.
- Installing physical barriers, such as clear plastic sneeze guards.

- Installing a drive-through window for customer service.
- Specialized negative pressure ventilation in some settings, such as for aerosol generating procedures (e.g., airborne infection isolation rooms in healthcare settings and specialized autopsy suites in mortuary settings).

Administrative Controls

Administrative controls require action by the worker or employer. Typically, administrative controls are changes in work policy or procedures to reduce or minimize exposure to a hazard. Examples of administrative controls for SARS-CoV-2 include:

- Encouraging sick workers to stay at home.
- Minimizing contact among workers, clients, and customers by replacing face-to-face meetings with virtual communications and implementing telework if feasible.
- Establishing alternating days or extra shifts that reduce the total number of employees in a facility at a given time, allowing them to maintain distance from one another while maintaining a full onsite work week.
- Discontinuing nonessential travel to locations with ongoing COVID-19 outbreaks. Regularly check CDC travel warning levels at: www.cdc.gov/coronavirus/2019-ncov/travelers.
- Developing emergency communications plans, including a forum for answering workers' concerns and internet-based communications, if feasible.
- Providing workers with up-to-date education and training on COVID-19 risk factors and protective behaviors (e.g., cough etiquette and care of PPE).
- Training workers who need to use protecting clothing and equipment how to put it on, use/wear it, and take it off correctly, including in the context of their current and potential duties. Training material should be easy to understand and available in the appropriate language and literacy level for all workers.

Safe Work Practices

Safe work practices are types of administrative controls that include procedures for safe and proper work used to reduce the duration, frequency, or intensity of exposure to a hazard. Examples of safe work practices for SARS-CoV-2 include:

- Providing resources and a work environment that promotes personal hygiene. For example, provide tissues, no-touch trash cans, hand soap, alcohol-based hand rubs containing at least 60 percent alcohol, disinfectants, and disposable towels for workers to clean their work surfaces.
- Requiring regular hand washing or using of alcohol-based hand rubs. Workers should always wash hands when they are visibly soiled and after removing any PPE.
- Post handwashing signs in restrooms.

Personal Protective Equipment (PPE)

While engineering and administrative controls are considered more effective in minimizing exposure to SARS-CoV-2, PPE may also be needed to prevent certain exposures. While correctly using PPE can help prevent some exposures, it should not take the place of other prevention strategies.

Examples of PPE include: gloves, goggles, face shields, face masks, and respiratory protection, when appropriate. During an outbreak of an infectious disease, such as COVID-19, recommendations for PPE specific to occupations or job tasks may change depending on geographic location, updated risk assessments for workers, and information on PPE effectiveness in preventing the spread of COVID-19. Employers should check the OSHA and CDC websites regularly for updates about recommended PPE.

All types of PPE must be:

- Selected based upon the hazard to the worker.
- Properly fitted and periodically refitted, as applicable (e.g., respirators).

- Consistently and properly worn when required.
- Regularly inspected, maintained, and replaced, as necessary.
- Properly removed, cleaned, and stored or disposed of, as applicable, to avoid contamination of self, others, or the environment.

Employers are obligated to provide their workers with PPE needed to keep them safe while performing their jobs. The types of PPE required during a COVID-19 outbreak will be based on the risk of being infected with SARS-CoV-2 while working and job tasks that may lead to exposure.

Workers, including those who work within 6 feet of patients known to be, or suspected of being, infected with SARS-CoV-2 and those performing aerosol-generating procedures, need to use respirators:

- National Institute for Occupational Safety and Health (NIOSH)-approved, N95 filtering facepiece respirators or better must be used in the context of a comprehensive, written respiratory protection program that includes fit-testing, training, and medical exams. See OSHA's Respiratory Protection standard, 29 CFR 1910.134 at www.osha.gov/laws-regs/regulations/standardnumber/1910/1910.134.
- When disposable N95 filtering facepiece respirators are not available, consider using other respirators that provide greater protection and improve worker comfort. Other types of acceptable respirators include: a R/P95, N/R/P99, or N/R/P100 filtering facepiece respirator; an air-purifying elastomeric (e.g., half-face or full-face) respirator with appropriate filters or cartridges; powered air purifying respirator (PAPR) with high-efficiency particulate arrestance (HEPA) filter; or supplied air respirator (SAR). See CDC/NIOSH guidance for optimizing respirator supplies at: www.cdc.gov/coronavirus/2019-ncov/hcp/respirators-strategy.

- Consider using PAPRs or SARs, which are more protective than filtering facepiece respirators, for any work operations or procedures likely to generate aerosols (e.g., cough induction procedures, some dental procedures, invasive specimen collection, blowing out pipettes, shaking or vortexing tubes, filling a syringe, centrifugation).

- Use a surgical N95 respirator when both respiratory protection and resistance to blood and body fluids is needed.

- Face shields may also be worn on top of a respirator to prevent bulk contamination of the respirator. Certain respirator designs with forward protrusions (duckbill style) may be difficult to properly wear under a face shield. Ensure that the face shield does not prevent airflow through the respirator.

- Consider factors such as function, fit, ability to decontaminate, disposal, and cost. OSHA's Respiratory Protection eTool provides basic information on respirators such as medical requirements, maintenance and care, fit testing, written respiratory protection programs, and voluntary use of respirators, which employers may also find beneficial in training workers at: www.osha.gov/SLTC/etools/respiratory. Also see NIOSH respirator guidance at: www.cdc.gov/niosh/topics/respirators.

- Respirator training should address selection, use (including donning and doffing), proper disposal or disinfection, inspection for damage, maintenance, and the limitations of respiratory protection equipment. Learn more at: www.osha.gov/SLTC/respiratoryprotection.

- The appropriate form of respirator will depend on the type of exposure and on the transmission pattern of COVID-19. See the NIOSH "Respirator Selection Logic" at: www.cdc.gov/niosh/docs/2005-100/default.html or the OSHA "Respiratory Protection eTool" at www.osha.gov/SLTC/etools/respiratory.

Follow Existing OSHA Standards

Existing OSHA standards may apply to protecting workers from exposure to and infection with SARS-CoV-2.

While there is no specific OSHA standard covering SARS-CoV-2 exposure, some OSHA requirements may apply to preventing occupational exposure to SARS-CoV-2. Among the most relevant are:

- OSHA's Personal Protective Equipment (PPE) standards (in general industry, 29 CFR 1910 Subpart I), which require using gloves, eye and face protection, and respiratory protection. See: www.osha.gov/laws-regs/regulations/standardnumber/1910#1910_Subpart_I.
  - When respirators are necessary to protect workers or where employers require respirator use, employers must implement a comprehensive respiratory protection program in accordance with the Respiratory Protection standard (29 CFR 1910.134). See: www.osha.gov/laws-regs/regulations/standardnumber/1910/1910.134.
- The General Duty Clause, Section 5(a)(1) of the Occupational Safety and Health (OSH) Act of 1970, 29 USC 654(a)(1), which requires employers to furnish to each worker "employment and a place of employment, which are free from recognized hazards that are causing or are likely to cause death or serious physical harm." See: www.osha.gov/laws-regs/oshact/completeoshact.

OSHA's Bloodborne Pathogens standard (29 CFR 1910.1030) applies to occupational exposure to human blood and other potentially infectious materials that typically do not include respiratory secretions that may transmit SARS-CoV-2. However, the provisions of the standard offer a framework that may help control some sources of the virus, including exposures to body fluids (e.g., respiratory secretions) not covered by the standard. See: www.osha.gov/laws-regs/regulations/standardnumber/1910/1910.1030.

The OSHA COVID-19 webpage provides additional information about OSHA standards and requirements, including requirements in states that operate their own OSHA-approved State Plans, recordkeeping requirements and injury/illness recording criteria, and applications of standards related to sanitation and communication of risks related to hazardous chemicals that may be in common sanitizers and sterilizers. See: www.osha.gov/SLTC/covid-19/standards.html.

Classifying Worker Exposure to SARS-CoV-2

Worker risk of occupational exposure to SARS-CoV-2, the virus that causes COVID-19, during an outbreak may vary from very high to high, medium, or lower (caution) risk. The level of risk depends in part on the industry type, need for contact within 6 feet of people known to be, or suspected of being, infected with SARS-CoV-2, or requirement for repeated or extended contact with persons known to be, or suspected of being, infected with SARS-CoV-2. To help employers determine appropriate precautions, OSHA has divided job tasks into four risk exposure levels: very high, high, medium, and lower risk. The Occupational Risk Pyramid shows the four exposure risk levels in the shape of a pyramid to represent probable distribution of risk. Most American workers will likely fall in the lower exposure risk (caution) or medium exposure risk levels.

**Occupational Risk Pyramid
for COVID-19**

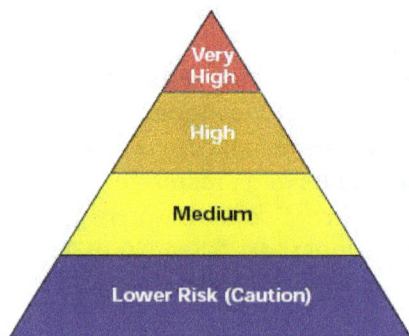

Very High Exposure Risk

Very high exposure risk jobs are those with high potential for exposure to known or suspected sources of COVID-19 during specific medical, postmortem, or laboratory procedures. Workers in this category include:

- Healthcare workers (e.g., doctors, nurses, dentists, paramedics, emergency medical technicians) performing aerosol-generating procedures (e.g., intubation, cough induction procedures, bronchoscopies, some dental procedures and exams, or invasive specimen collection) on known or suspected COVID-19 patients.
- Healthcare or laboratory personnel collecting or handling specimens from known or suspected COVID-19 patients (e.g., manipulating cultures from known or suspected COVID-19 patients).
- Morgue workers performing autopsies, which generally involve aerosol-generating procedures, on the bodies of people who are known to have, or suspected of having, COVID-19 at the time of their death.

High Exposure Risk

High exposure risk jobs are those with high potential for exposure to known or suspected sources of COVID-19. Workers in this category include:

- Healthcare delivery and support staff (e.g., doctors, nurses, and other hospital staff who must enter patients' rooms) exposed to known or suspected COVID-19 patients. (Note: when such workers perform aerosol-generating procedures, their exposure risk level becomes *very high.*)
- Medical transport workers (e.g., ambulance vehicle operators) moving known or suspected COVID-19 patients in enclosed vehicles.
- Mortuary workers involved in preparing (e.g., for burial or cremation) the bodies of people who are known to have, or suspected of having, COVID-19 at the time of their death.

Medium Exposure Risk

Medium exposure risk jobs include those that require frequent and/or close contact with (i.e., within 6 feet of) people who may be infected with SARS-CoV-2, but who are not known or suspected COVID-19 patients. In areas without ongoing community transmission, workers in this risk group may have frequent contact with travelers who may return from international locations with widespread COVID-19 transmission. In areas where there *is* ongoing community transmission, workers in this category may have contact with the general public (e.g., schools, high-population-density work environments, some high-volume retail settings).

Lower Exposure Risk (Caution)

Lower exposure risk (caution) jobs are those that do not require contact with people known to be, or suspected of being, infected with SARS-CoV-2 nor frequent close contact with (i.e., within 6 feet of) the general public. Workers in this category have minimal occupational contact with the public and other coworkers.

Jobs Classified at Lower Exposure Risk (Caution): What to Do to Protect Workers

For workers who do not have frequent contact with the general public, employers should follow the guidance for "Steps All Employers Can Take to Reduce Workers' Risk of Exposure to SARS-CoV-2," on page 7 of this booklet and implement control measures described in this section.

Engineering Controls

Additional engineering controls are not recommended for workers in the lower exposure risk group. Employers should ensure that engineering controls, if any, used to protect workers from other job hazards continue to function as intended.

Administrative Controls

- Monitor public health communications about COVID-19 recommendations and ensure that workers have access to that information. Frequently check the CDC COVID-19 website: www.cdc.gov/coronavirus/2019-ncov.
- Collaborate with workers to designate effective means of communicating important COVID-19 information.

Personal Protective Equipment

Additional PPE is not recommended for workers in the lower exposure risk group. Workers should continue to use the PPE, if any, that they would ordinarily use for other job tasks.

Jobs Classified at Medium Exposure Risk: What to Do to Protect Workers

In workplaces where workers have medium exposure risk, employers should follow the guidance for "Steps All Employers Can Take to Reduce Workers' Risk of Exposure to SARS-CoV-2," on page 7 of this booklet and implement control measures described in this section.

Engineering Controls

- Install physical barriers, such as clear plastic sneeze guards, where feasible.

Administrative Controls

- Consider offering face masks to ill employees and customers to contain respiratory secretions until they are able leave the workplace (i.e., for medical evaluation/care or to return home). In the event of a shortage of masks, a reusable face shield that can be decontaminated may be an acceptable method of protecting against droplet transmission. See CDC/ NIOSH guidance for optimizing respirator supplies, which discusses the use of surgical masks, at: www.cdc.gov/ coronavirus/2019-ncov/hcp/respirators-strategy.

- Keep customers informed about symptoms of COVID-19 and ask sick customers to minimize contact with workers until healthy again, such as by posting signs about COVID-19 in stores where sick customers may visit (e.g., pharmacies) or including COVID-19 information in automated messages sent when prescriptions are ready for pick up.
- Where appropriate, limit customers' and the public's access to the worksite, or restrict access to only certain workplace areas.
- Consider strategies to minimize face-to-face contact (e.g., drive-through windows, phone-based communication, telework).
- Communicate the availability of medical screening or other worker health resources (e.g., on-site nurse; telemedicine services).

Personal Protective Equipment (PPE)

When selecting PPE, consider factors such as function, fit, decontamination ability, disposal, and cost. Sometimes, when PPE will have to be used repeatedly for a long period of time, a more expensive and durable type of PPE may be less expensive overall than disposable PPE. Each employer should select the combination of PPE that protects workers specific to their workplace.

Workers with medium exposure risk may need to wear some combination of gloves, a gown, a face mask, and/or a face shield or goggles. PPE ensembles for workers in the medium exposure risk category will vary by work task, the results of the employer's hazard assessment, and the types of exposures workers have on the job.

High exposure risk jobs are those with high potential for exposure to known or suspected sources of COVID-19.

Very high exposure risk jobs are those with high potential for exposure to known or suspected sources of COVID-19 during specific medical, postmortem, or laboratory procedures that involve aerosol generation or specimen collection/handling.

In rare situations that would require workers in this risk category to use respirators, see the PPE section beginning on page 14 of this booklet, which provides more details about respirators. For the most up-to-date information, visit OSHA's COVID-19 webpage: www.osha.gov/covid-19.

Jobs Classified at High or Very High Exposure Risk: What to Do to Protect Workers

In workplaces where workers have high or very high exposure risk, employers should follow the guidance for "Steps All Employers Can Take to Reduce Workers' Risk of Exposure to SARS-CoV-2," on page 7 of this booklet and implement control measures described in this section.

Engineering Controls

- Ensure appropriate air-handling systems are installed and maintained in healthcare facilities. See "Guidelines for Environmental Infection Control in Healthcare Facilities" for more recommendations on air handling systems at: www. cdc.gov/mmwr/preview/mmwrhtml/rr5210a1.htm.

- CDC recommends that patients with known or suspected COVID-19 (i.e., person under investigation) should be placed in an airborne infection isolation room (AIIR), if available.

- Use isolation rooms when available for performing aerosol-generating procedures on patients with known or suspected COVID-19. For postmortem activities, use autopsy suites or other similar isolation facilities when performing aerosol-generating procedures on the bodies of people who are known to have, or suspected of having, COVID-19 at the time of their death. See the CDC postmortem guidance at: www.cdc.gov/coronavirus/2019-ncov/hcp/guidance-postmortem-specimens.html. OSHA also provides guidance for postmortem activities on its COVID-19 webpage: www.osha.gov/covid-19.

- Use special precautions associated with Biosafety Level 3 when handling specimens from known or suspected COVID-19 patients. For more information about biosafety levels, consult the U.S. Department of Health and Human Services (HHS) "Biosafety in Microbiological and Biomedical Laboratories" at www.cdc.gov/biosafety/publications/bmbl5.

Administrative Controls

If working in a healthcare facility, follow existing guidelines and facility standards of practice for identifying and isolating infected individuals and for protecting workers.

- Develop and implement policies that reduce exposure, such as cohorting (i.e., grouping) COVID-19 patients when single rooms are not available.
- Post signs requesting patients and family members to immediately report symptoms of respiratory illness on arrival at the healthcare facility and use disposable face masks.
- Consider offering enhanced medical monitoring of workers during COVID-19 outbreaks.
- Provide all workers with job-specific education and training on preventing transmission of COVID-19, including initial and routine/refresher training.
- Ensure that psychological and behavioral support is available to address employee stress.

Safe Work Practices

- Provide emergency responders and other essential personnel who may be exposed while working away from fixed facilities with alcohol-based hand rubs containing at least 60% alcohol for decontamination in the field.

Personal Protective Equipment (PPE)

Most workers at high or very high exposure risk likely need to wear gloves, a gown, a face shield or goggles, and either a face mask or a respirator, depending on their job tasks and exposure risks.

Those who work closely with (either in contact with or within 6 feet of) patients known to be, or suspected of being, infected with SARS-CoV-2, the virus that causes COVID-19, should wear respirators. In these instances, see the PPE section beginning on page 14 of this booklet, which provides more details about respirators. For the most up-to-date information, also visit OSHA's COVID-19 webpage: www.osha.gov/covid-19.

PPE ensembles may vary, especially for workers in laboratories or morgue/mortuary facilities who may need additional protection against blood, body fluids, chemicals, and other materials to which they may be exposed. Additional PPE may include medical/surgical gowns, fluid-resistant coveralls, aprons, or other disposable or reusable protective clothing. Gowns should be large enough to cover the areas requiring protection. OSHA may also provide updated guidance for PPE use on its website: www.osha.gov/covid-19.

NOTE: Workers who dispose of PPE and other infectious waste must also be trained and provided with appropriate PPE.

The CDC webpage "Healthcare-associated Infections" (www.cdc.gov/hai) provides additional information on infection control in healthcare facilities.

Workers Living Abroad or Travelling Internationally

Employers with workers living abroad or traveling on international business should consult the "Business Travelers" section of the OSHA COVID-19 webpage (www.osha.gov/covid-19), which also provides links to the latest:

- CDC travel warnings: www.cdc.gov/coronavirus/2019-ncov/travelers
- U.S. Department of State (DOS) travel advisories: travel.state.gov

Employers should communicate to workers that the DOS cannot provide Americans traveling or living abroad with medications or supplies, even in the event of a COVID-19 outbreak.

As COVID-19 outbreak conditions change, travel into or out of a country may not be possible, safe, or medically advisable. It is also likely that governments will respond to a COVID-19 outbreak by imposing public health measures that restrict domestic and international movement, further limiting the U.S. government's ability to assist Americans in these countries. It is important that employers and workers plan appropriately, as it is possible that these measures will be implemented very quickly in the event of worsening outbreak conditions in certain areas.

More information on COVID-19 planning for workers living and traveling abroad can be found at: www.cdc.gov/travel.

For More Information

Federal, state, and local government agencies are the best source of information in the event of an infectious disease outbreak, such as COVID-19. Staying informed about the latest developments and recommendations is critical, since specific guidance may change based upon evolving outbreak situations.

Below are several recommended websites to access the most current and accurate information:

- Occupational Safety and Health Administration website: www.osha.gov
- Centers for Disease Control and Prevention website: www.cdc.gov
- National Institute for Occupational Safety and Health website: www.cdc.gov/niosh

OSHA Assistance, Services, and Programs

OSHA has a great deal of information to assist employers in complying with their responsibilities under OSHA law. Several OSHA programs and services can help employers identify and correct job hazards, as well as improve their safety and health program.

Establishing a Safety and Health Program

Safety and health programs are systems that can substantially reduce the number and severity of workplace injuries and illnesses, while reducing costs to employers.

Visit www.osha.gov/safetymanagement for more information.

Compliance Assistance Specialists

OSHA compliance assistance specialists can provide information to employers and workers about OSHA standards, short educational programs on specific hazards or OSHA rights and responsibilities, and information on additional compliance assistance resources.

Visit www.osha.gov/complianceassistance/cas or call 1-800-321-OSHA (6742) to contact your local OSHA office.

No-Cost On-Site Safety and Health Consultation Services for Small Business

OSHA's On-Site Consultation Program offers no-cost and confidential advice to small and medium-sized businesses in all states, with priority given to high-hazard worksites. On-Site consultation services are separate from enforcement and do not result in penalties or citations.

For more information or to find the local On-Site Consultation office in your state, visit www.osha.gov/consultation, or call 1-800-321-OSHA (6742).

Under the consultation program, certain exemplary employers may request participation in OSHA's **Safety and Health Achievement Recognition Program (SHARP)**. Worksites that receive SHARP recognition are exempt from programmed inspections during the period that the SHARP certification is valid.

Cooperative Programs

OSHA offers cooperative programs under which businesses, labor groups and other organizations can work cooperatively with OSHA. To find out more about any of the following programs, visit www.osha.gov/cooperativeprograms.

Strategic Partnerships and Alliances

The OSHA Strategic Partnerships (OSP) provide the opportunity for OSHA to partner with employers, workers, professional or trade associations, labor organizations, and/or other interested stakeholders. Through the Alliance Program, OSHA works with groups to develop compliance assistance tools and resources to share with workers and employers, and educate workers and employers about their rights and responsibilities.

Voluntary Protection Programs (VPP)

The VPP recognize employers and workers in the private sector and federal agencies who have implemented effective safety and health programs and maintain injury and illness rates below the national average for their respective industries.

Occupational Safety and Health Training

OSHA partners with 26 OSHA Training Institute Education Centers at 37 locations throughout the United States to deliver courses on OSHA standards and occupational safety and health topics to thousands of students a year. For more information on training courses, visit www.osha.gov/otiec.

OSHA Educational Materials

OSHA has many types of educational materials to assist employers and workers in finding and preventing workplace hazards.

All OSHA publications are free at www.osha.gov/publications and www.osha.gov/ebooks. You can also call 1-800-321-OSHA (6742) to order publications.

Employers and safety and health professionals can sign-up for *QuickTakes*, OSHA's free, twice-monthly online newsletter with the latest news about OSHA initiatives and products to assist in finding and preventing workplace hazards. To sign up, visit www.osha.gov/quicktakes.

OSHA Regional Offices

Region 1
Boston Regional Office
(CT*, ME*, MA, NH, RI, VT*)
JFK Federal Building
25 New Sudbury Street, Room E340
Boston, MA 02203
(617) 565-9860 (617) 565-9827 Fax

Region 2
New York Regional Office
(NJ*, NY*, PR*, VI*)
Federal Building
201 Varick Street, Room 670
New York, NY 10014
(212) 337-2378 (212) 337-2371 Fax

Region 3
Philadelphia Regional Office
(DE, DC, MD*, PA, VA*, WV)
The Curtis Center
170 S. Independence Mall West, Suite 740 West
Philadelphia, PA 19106-3309
(215) 861-4900 (215) 861-4904 Fax

Region 4
Atlanta Regional Office
(AL, FL, GA, KY*, MS, NC*, SC*, TN*)
Sam Nunn Atlanta Federal Center
61 Forsyth Street, SW, Room 6T50
Atlanta, GA 30303
(678) 237-0400 (678) 237-0447 Fax

Region 5
Chicago Regional Office
(IL*, IN*, MI*, MN*, OH, WI)
John C. Kluczynski Federal Building
230 South Dearborn Street, Room 3244
Chicago, IL 60604
(312) 353-2220 (312) 353-7774 Fax

Region 6
Dallas Regional Office
(AR, LA, NM*, OK, TX)
A. Maceo Smith Federal Building
525 Griffin Street, Room 602
Dallas, TX 75202
(972) 850-4145 (972) 850-4149 Fax

Region 7
Kansas City Regional Office
(IA*, KS, MO, NE)
Two Pershing Square Building
2300 Main Street, Suite 1010
Kansas City, MO 64108-2416
(816) 283-8745 (816) 283-0547 Fax

Region 8
Denver Regional Office
(CO, MT, ND, SD, UT*, WY*)
Cesar Chavez Memorial Building
1244 Speer Boulevard, Suite 551
Denver, CO 80204
(720) 264-6550 (720) 264-6585 Fax

Region 9

San Francisco Regional Office
(AZ*, CA*, HI*, NV*, and American Samoa,
Guam and the Northern Mariana Islands)
San Francisco Federal Building
90 7th Street, Suite 2650
San Francisco, CA 94103
(415) 625-2547 (415) 625-2534 Fax

Region 10

Seattle Regional Office
(AK*, ID, OR*, WA*)
Fifth & Yesler Tower
300 Fifth Avenue, Suite 1280
Seattle, WA 98104
(206) 757-6700 (206) 757-6705 Fax

*These states and territories operate their own OSHA-approved job safety and health plans and cover state and local government employees as well as private sector employees. The Connecticut, Illinois, Maine, New Jersey, New York and Virgin Islands programs cover public employees only. (Private sector workers in these states are covered by Federal OSHA). States with approved programs must have standards that are identical to, or at least as effective as, the Federal OSHA standards.

Note: To get contact information for OSHA area offices, OSHA-approved state plans and OSHA consultation projects, please visit us online at www.osha.gov or call us at 1-800-321-OSHA (6742).

How to Contact OSHA

Under the Occupational Safety and Health Act of 1970, employers are responsible for providing safe and healthful workplaces for their employees. OSHA's role is to help ensure these conditions for America's working men and women by setting and enforcing standards, and providing training, education and assistance. For more information, visit www.osha.gov or call OSHA at 1-800-321-OSHA (6742), TTY 1-877-889-5627.

**For assistance, contact us.
We are OSHA. We can help.**

OSHA®
www.osha.gov